Swinging For Couples Vol. 1

Beginner's Guide To The Swinging
Lifestyle - 25 Things You Must Know
Before Becoming A Swinger

Natalie Robinson

Swinging For Couples Vol. 1

Publisher: Enlightened Publishing

ISBN-13: 978-1518652981

ISBN-10: 1518652980

Disclaimer

The Publisher has strived to be as accurate and complete as possible in the creation of this book. While all attempts have been made to verify information provided in this publication, the Publisher assumes no responsibility for errors, omissions, or contrary interpretation of the subject matter herein. Any perceived slights of specific persons, peoples, or organizations are unintentional.

This book is not intended for use as a source of legal, business, accounting or financial advice. All readers are advised to seek services of competent professionals in the legal, business, accounting, and finance fields.

The information in this book is not intended or implied to be a substitute for professional medical advice, diagnosis or treatment. All content contained in this book is for general information purposes only. Always consult your healthcare provider before carrying on any health program.

Table of Contents

Introduction 5

Terms and Acronyms 9

Chapter 1: Self-esteem and Self-confidence in a
Swinging Relationship 17

   #1. Know Yourself and Be Confident 18

   #2. Express Yourself and Your Desires 21

   #3. Open Your Mind 27

   #4. Have Fun 30

Chapter 2: Maintaining a Healthy Relationship
While Swinging 35

   #5. Do – Have a solid, healthy, honest, and
communicative relationship before
swinging. 36

   #6. Don't – Do this to "fix" a broken
relationship. 39

   #7. Do – Talk about sex............................... 42

   #8. Don't – Assume anything about your
partner or their expectations. 45

#9. Do – Know each other's boundaries very well and discuss what would happen should these boundaries be crossed... 47

#10. Don't – Push those boundaries. This will guarantee failure............................. 49

Chapter 3: Communication and Following the Rules.. 51

#11. Know the Rules..................................... 51

#12. Communication between You and Your Partner... 55

#13. Communication between Two Swinging Couples 57

#14. Communication in Various Club Environments and Private Parties 58

Chapter 4: Meeting Other Swingers............... 61

#15. Meeting Swingers Online.................... 62

#16. Meeting Swingers at Off-site Clubs and Events... 67

#17. Meeting Swingers at On-site Clubs and Parties.. 68

#18. Joining a Private Swingers' Club........ 69

Chapter 5: You Are at the Party, Now What?
.... 73

#19. Take the Pressure Off of Your First
    Time Out.. 73

#20. Breaking the Ice 74

#21. Smile... 75

#22. Dance.. 76

#23. Socialize 79

#24. Don't Be Shy.. 80

#25. Have Fun! 82

Conclusion 85

Introduction

So you think you are ready to swing? Perhaps you've heard about swinging from some friends, seen a reality show about swinging, or read about it online. Possibly, your significant other has been talking about it. You've thought about it, and it sounds interesting, fun, and sexy, but how exactly does swinging work? What are the options? Are there rules? Where do you meet other swingers?

Fortunately, you have come to the right place. This introductory book will guide you through the basics of swinging for couples.

Swinging has been growing more popular in the last few years, as more options have become available for like-minded individuals to connect. Swinging may seem like a new concept to you, but the truth is that people have been engaging in this activity for a long time. Different societies and cultures, from Europe to South America to Africa, have practiced a form of partner swapping for as long as there have been people having sex.

In North America and Europe, there was a small, but active, swinger's movement in the 1970's. Swinging has made a large comeback over the past five to ten years, even gaining momentum in more mainstream society.

Once you start exploring the idea of swinging, you'll be surprised at who else is swinging, and how many different walks of life are involved in this activity. From older, established, professional couples to younger, less experienced couples, everyone shares in the same passion and goal of having fun and pursuing a new level of sexual satisfaction.

There are many couples and partners out there who share themselves not only with each other, but also with other adults who share their sexual enthusiasm. Most people swing with class, grace, and discretion. Many would say that they experience amazing results when they bring their sexual desires and fantasies to life.

This lifestyle has room for almost everyone, provided that you enter into it with respect and open-mindedness towards your fellow swingers and their sometimes odd quirks and fetishes. There is a wonderful world waiting for you and your partner, which should include a happy relationship, great friends, and amazing sexual adventures, if you know the right path to take.

Most sexual interactions have the nature of being discreet and "hush-hush," so it is one-hundred percent natural to feel as though getting into a swingers' club might be harder than getting into an Ivy League school. Rest assured. Finding fellow swingers is nowhere near this hard. As long as you go about it with knowledge, confidence, and a great partner, swinging is a not a daunting task at all, but a very enjoyable experience for everyone. Take the time to educate yourself and your partner before you begin this amazing and sexy journey together.

Ready? Let's get started.

Terms and Acronyms

The journey towards swinging starts with an understanding of some of the lingo used, not only throughout this book, but also throughout the swinging lifestyle. These are important for interacting with other couples, both online and in person.

This section covers the basic and general terms. Although not an exhaustive list, it is a good place to start. Being familiar with these terms will not only help online forums or fetish conversations make more sense, but also allow you to communicate your needs and desires more clearly with other swinging couples.

- **AC/DC**: This is another way to say someone is bisexual.

- **On-Site vs. Off-Site Clubs**: An on-site club or party is one that allows sexual intercourse and public displays of affection. Some events allow for public playing, while others have rooms set aside for more intimate relations to be had separately.

An off-site club or event is one that does not allow public sexual relations. The couples who wish to interact intimately with each other must arrange for such events to take place off premise at their own home, hotel room, or other agreed upon meeting place.

- **Full Swap vs. Soft Swap**: A full swap occurs when two (at least) couples switch partners for the purpose of sex. This can include oral only, full penetration, or both, depending on the limits of all involved.

A soft swap entails having sex with another couple in the room, but usually there is no swapping of partners. If there is a swapping, it may entail oral sex only, or some other activity that is short of actual penetration.

- **Closed Swinging vs. Open Swinging**: Closed swinging occurs when the partners of each couple swap and have sex in separate beds and rooms, often with closed doors. This is also referred to as different-room swap.

Open swinging entails the partners swapping with all four people on the same bed or in the same room during the sex and playtime.

- **Playtime or Playing**: Playtime or playing refers to having sex or foreplay.

- **Bareback**: Having sexual intercourse without the protection of a condom.

- **Bisexual vs Bicomfortable vs Bicouple**: A bisexual is a person who enjoys sexual contact with both sexes. Such a person can also be referred to as Bi or AC/DC.

A bicomfortable person is someone who is comfortable being around another person who is bisexual, and open to participating in multi-person group sex, although not comfortable giving oral sex or kissing people of the same sex. Some bicomfortable people are comfortable receiving sexual attention from the same sex but not with giving it. Be sure to clarify before entering into the bedroom with them.

A bicouple is a couple in which both partners are bisexual.

- **Anal Sex**: The act of a penis or toy penetrating one's anus. "**Greek**" is one term that refers to anal sex, and "**the backdoor**" is another reference to one's anus. "**Brown eye**" and "**corn hole**" are cruder terms that are also used to reference the anus (as is of course the word "asshole").

- **Double Penetration**: Double penetration occurs when the woman has both her vagina and asshole filled by either two cocks, two toys, or one of each, and is often referred to as DP. Double penetration can be administered by men or women or with toys. **DAP** is double anal penetration and **DVP** is double vaginal penetration.

- **Air-tight**: One step past double penetration, where the woman also has a
  cock in her mouth.

- **Orgy**: An orgy is sex between multiple
  partners or more than four people sim-
  ultaneously. It is also referred to as
  "Roman" from time to time, as the Ro-
  mans were known to have been very
  promiscuous and comfortable with
  group sex.

- **French**: This term is often used to refer
  to oral sex, but can be used to describe
  the style of kissing as well.

- **Permission Slips and Hall Passes**:
  Permission slips and hall passes are
  granted to one half or both halves of the
  couple when one of the partners is going to be away from the other. The parameters of the passes can vary from
  couple to couple. These usually allow
  the holder of the hall pass or permission slip to have intimate relations with
  someone else while their partners are
  away.

- **C2C**: C2C stands for Cam to Cam, and is important to know for when other couples want to cam chat with you. This is a very fun and erotic experience, and a great way, especially for new swingers, to feel out your compatibility with another couple.

- **BBC**: This acronym means Big Black Cock and is a term that usually references interracial sex.

- **BBW**: Big Beautiful Woman (or women) and can sometimes mean Big Black Woman.

- **B&D**: Bondage & Discipline, which includes discipline and power games and roles, as well as binding and restricting a person during sexual play.

- **BDSM**: The fetish of Bondage and Discipline, Dominance and Submission, Sadism and Masochism. Very similar to B&D, it includes the aspect of deriving sexual pleasure from pain, as well as being disciplined, tied up, and bound.

- **Vanilla**: In a swinger's world, vanilla refers to couples who do not swing, and people who are not in the lifestyle or have yet become introduced fully to it. It can also be the antithesis of "kinky." In some circles this is a derogatory term.

Chapter 1: Self-esteem and Self-confidence in a Swinging Relationship

The importance of self-esteem and self-confidence in a swinging relationship cannot be stressed enough. Most of us heard about the importance of loving ourselves and how it will help us live a balanced life. Self-confidence is just as crucial to the swinger life-style as it is to any lifestyle.

Within self-confidence lies the ability which allows us to clearly, consistently, and healthily communicate with others in our life. When you have confidence in yourself, you have the ability to be confident as a couple as well.

No matter who else is around us, or what their ideas or values are, self-confidence gives us the power to hold true to our own values and ideas. Simply put, it allows us to interact with an open-mind with others without changing or losing faith in our own beliefs and behaviors.

Finally, and most importantly, being in tune with one's self and one's confidence enables us to be happy and have fun in many aspects of life. This is no doubt the most helpful trait to possess when approaching swinging.

#1. Know Yourself and Be Confident

Don't fret that this is going to turn into a self-help book. It is important, however, to know why knowing yourself and being self-confident matters, and how it will help you on your journey to becoming a successful swinger.

Jealousy can easily abound within the swinging environment if left unchecked, but it does not have to be present in your experience, as long as you maintain confidence in both yourself and your relationships. Can you imagine a room full of insecure women (or men, for that matter) picking at each other? It would feel more like high school instead of a sexy social scene with beautiful confident adults involved.

If you are the type of person who picks themselves apart because your friend looks cuter than you in those shorts, then I highly doubt that it is going to work out very well when you are in bed together with each other's husbands (or wives). Be comfortable enough in your own skin that you actually love it. Do not let yourself compare your body to someone else's, but rather appreciate them all for their own unique beauty. We are all beautiful and sexy in our own different ways. Comparing and degrading yourself or others is not the way to have a fun and sexy night.

This is why self-confidence and self-love are so important. If you love yourself and appreciate your own beauty, you will be able to let go of comparing and judging other bodies around you. You will learn to love them and enjoy them for who and what their sexy selves are. Enjoy the beauty of diversity and differences and love the things that make you and others unique. If we all looked the same, things would get a bit boring after a while. It is important to celebrate loving yourself, your body, your thoughts, and opinions.

Be sure to know and love your sexual self as well. Know what you like and what you don't. Know what you are and are not attracted to as a couple. Are you straight, bisexual, or bicurious? Know what you are willing to experiment with, and what you are not.

The longer you are in the swingers' world, the more you will face just about anything and everything. Some people enjoy some light BDSM, and some prefer heavier aspects of that activity, while others don't like it at all. Fetishes can range from water sports to foot fetishes, so be ready to say yes or no to just about anything.

Prepare yourself by knowing what you want as a couple and individuals. This is critical to enjoying yourself sexually during a playdate or party. Spend a lot of time thinking about these things and knowing what you want. Talk about it with your partner or your close friends.

If there are certain things you wish to try, but not with a stranger, try it out with your partner first. The point is to know and love yourself, your partner, your body, their bodies, and each other's thoughts and opinions. The rest will fall into place easily.

#2. Express Yourself and Your Desires

Being able to confidently express yourself is another character trait that is imperative to the swinging process. Just as in personal relationships, work, and normal social interactions, the better you can communicate confidently with other people, the more you are able to work productively together. Communication works the same way in the swinging lifestyle. To be able to comfortably and confidently express these desires not only to your partner but also to other swinging couples is critical.

Have honest conversations about what you are or are not comfortable with sexually as couples. Talk about what you are comfortable doing sexually with others, as well as what you are comfortable being around and watching together. Are you open to clubs and parties where play is public, and there is group playtime? Or do the two of you prefer a more intimate and discreet setting and swapping scenario? Setting up a successful swinging encounter for the two of you rests largely on your ability to know and express your own desires as a couple.

Have the confidence to not only express consent but also to say no if you feel like it. Don't ever go into a situation to have sex with people in a way in which you are not comfortable. Nor should you have sex with people you are not attracted to because of inability to tell your partner or another couple no, or because you were not confident enough to speak up. You will feel terrible, and it almost always causes pent-up resentment or emotional hostility.

Not only is expressing yourself important to your own sexual health and relationship with your partner, but it is also a critical element when interacting with other swingers. If you can't talk to your partner about sex, you will certainly have a problem talking about it to couples you just meet.

Being able to tell your partner exactly what you want will lead to the two of you being closer, as well as to avoid terrible confusion and hurt later on. It is much easier to say, "I'd be willing to try anal with you, baby, but we need to go slow. I'm scared that it will hurt," than to say, "Ok, let's do it," and grimace, bear it, and have a miserable anal experience.

Summon the confidence to bring up the subject and say exactly how you feel about the situation. You could start out with, "I'm willing to try but every time I've done it in the past, it hurt really badly." A smart, receptive partner will listen and respond with options and kindness: "What would make you enjoy it more? Did they use lube on you or play with you first, or did they just try to stick it in?"

The more you discuss sex with your partner and with other couples, the easier it will become. Most men and women aren't used to expressing their personal sexual desires and fantasies. These feelings are usually private, and we aren't quite sure how other people will react. Perhaps you told someone in the past and were open about what you wished for but only to have your feelings hurt or be treated carelessly. Surprisingly, a lot of bad sexual experiences come from one or two poor encounters with some unfortunate, uneducated sop who knows very little about proper sex.

All the above makes it hard to discuss your sexual desires with other people, especially with the person that you are closest to. A great way to overcome all that is to interact with a group of wonderfully open-minded adults who are looking for sexual adventure as well. When you discuss your thoughts and feelings with other swingers, you will find that the conversation, while honest, is light-hearted and non-judgmental. If someone has different wants or desires that you don't agree with, simply continue talking to people and getting to know them until you do find someone who meshes well with your personal style.

Be ready to talk about a variety of sexually charged situations for both partners, from bi-sexuality, transgender, and homosexual situations to sexually transmitted diseases (STDs) and pregnancy prevention. Discuss what the boundaries and limitations will be (if there are any) with other couples.

Some questions you and your partner should know the answers to include:

- Will you allow oral sex?

- Will you allow anal sex?

- Are you interested in full penetration or just sex play?

- Are you interested in having sex with the other couples in the same room or would you prefer to separate and rejoin later?

- Do you just want to watch while your significant other having sex?

- How involved do you want to be?

- Is either of you bisexual or bi-curious? If so, are you wanting to explore?

Regardless of whether or not either of the partners is bisexual, the parameters of full swap vs. soft swap and other playing rules should be determined and clarified prior to entering into any tryst with another couple.

For the couples who have a bisexual partner, the options become a bit more numerous, and there are a few more things that need to be discussed.

For Bisexual Partners

The idea of having a bisexual partner can be thrilling or scary depending on who you are. Whichever way you feel, be honest about it with your partner. If you are terrified of the thought, but still into swinging, then a closed swap would likely be more attractive to you than all four of you playing together.

Many men who have a bisexual female partner have found that one of their dreams has finally come true. The man who is not into such interactions can still allow his partner to fulfill her needs and desires by letting her play with other couples or just other ladies.

I highly suggest that if you have a bisexual partner, do not try to prevent them from having same sex lovers. This can lead to resentment, especially if the two of you are in sexually charged situations often. The point of swinging is not to restrain your partner but for you two to find your truest and freest sexual selves. If you are not bicomfortable or bisexual, then let them play with others in close, soft swap exchanges. The above advice holds true for women who are in relationships with bisexual men.

For those who enjoy the thought of having a bisexual lover, keep the expectations of these encounters realistic and be prepared to not be the center of attention. One could even find that they and the other partner are on the sidelines watching the two same sex partners making love while they are being left out. Ideally you will roll with the punches and be involved when the opportunity presents itself. Even more ideal, you will have talked about all of these situations, so you know what to expect from each other and remain realistic.

When you do find yourself in a threesome, enjoy the attention when it is focused on you, and give attention to at least one, if not both, of the other lovers when it is not. If you are in the position of being able to play with them both, be sure to pay an equal amount of attention and time to the best of your ability, unless of course you and your partner have discussed otherwise.

Follow all of the rules that you have set up between each other and for the other party or couple involved. Each couple and interaction can be different, so discuss parameters not only with your partner but also with the other couple before things go too far.

#3. Open Your Mind

Swinging is a lifestyle created by open-minded people for other open-minded people. It is especially appealing to adults who love to have fun and are open to different fetishes and sexual trysts, ranging from Dominance and submission, to role-playing, voyeurism, and exhibitionism.

You will find some swingers that want to have sex without their partners anywhere around. You will find couples that will only have sex with other couples at the same time. There are those who prefer group sex, and women and men who lust for multiple couples while their partners watch. There are women who like to have sex with other women, and there are husbands and wives who don't even want to touch another woman. It is not unusual to encounter slaves and Masters, men with multiple female partners, and the occasional girl who is looking for a couple to take her in. The longer you swing, the more you will see, experience, and witness.

This is not a lifestyle for close-minded people. This is a lifestyle for people who want to have fun, learn, and try new things, as well as for those who aren't afraid to see what sexual adventures and excitement await them. If there are certain aspects of sexuality that are not appealing to a certain couple, they must still be comfortable with that being the style for somebody else, even if they choose not to partake.

At parties, clubs, meet and greets, events, or even just chatting with other swingers online, new swinging couples are exposed to different levels of nudity, as well as very frank and honest discussions about sex. Learn to listen to the ideas, wants, and desires of your partner and those around you that are willing to talk about them.

Find out what different people's quirks and fetishes are. If those quirks and fetishes are not for you, don't worry about it. Learn to have fun with new people, talk and get to know them. Hanging out and being social at swinger events is key. Even if you are not swapping with the couple, you can still have an interesting conversation and get to know them as friends.

If a couple is not open to the different sexual tastes and preferences of others, they are diminishing their chances of finding a couple who is open to their own tastes and preferences. Being open-minded does not mean that couples will sleep together only if they have the same preferences and tastes. It does mean that they are able to hold a friendly, polite, and fun conversation with the other couple in an attempt to get to know them and find out if they are compatible. At some point, the couples can agree that they make a good fit, or move on to meeting and getting to know others in hopes of finding a more compatible match. As long as you maintain an open-mind you will find that others will be more open to you.

#4. Have Fun

This might seem obvious, but seriously everyone, swinging is about having fun! Enjoy yourself and your partner, party, dance, and make wonderful new and fascinating friends, explore your sexual fantasies like you've never dreamed you could. If this does not sound fun to you, and you are doing it only to please your partner or for some other reason, then you need to rethink your choice to explore swinging.

It is so easy to get caught up in impressing other people or acting like the "Joneses" of the Swinging World. Don't fall into the trap of being wrapped up in the mission of finding another couple to play with, or focusing so much on the search that you forget to enjoy yourselves. This can cause you to miss out on the fun.

Remember, swinging is a journey-driven process, not a goal-driven process. Journey-driven processes are motivated and propelled by the joy of the journey itself. It is a process that is pleasurable, exciting, and memorable the whole way through. People who are on an adventure, and are confident in themselves, enjoy journey-driven processes and will make the most of them.

Swinging can be one of the greatest adventures of your life, if you learn to kick back, relax, and have fun. Be prepared to make new friends with whom you can share a level of candid honesty unparalleled to the relationships built at work or in other aspects of your life. The beauty about focusing on having fun instead of having lots of sex is that the lots of sex part follows the fun part very quickly. Everyone would rather hang out with a smiling, laughing, and happy person than a brooding, quiet, and mysterious one on a mission to get laid.

Having fun includes, but not limited to, dancing, having witty conversations with others, mingling, teasing and joking, light tickling, and even having conversations that have nothing to do with sex. You don't have to start tickling strangers right off the bat, but I do suggest doing this with your partner. Playful pinches, grabs, and rubs always help to get the mood going. The more you do this to each other and lighten the mood, the more others will respond and are more likely to join you.

Have fun with your clothes on as well as off. I once went to a swinger's party where the birthday girl was wearing nothing but a "dress" made out of balloons. As each couple and guest came in, they got to pick a balloon off of her dress. It did not take long for the men and women at the party to begin using those balloons creatively. Some were playing with balloons as breasts and balls, joking around, and holding them against each other. Pretty soon the ladies had their shirts off and were playfully comparing the balloons to each other's breasts and drawing nipples on the balloons.

It was silly and fun and really got everyone interacting with each other comfortably. It broke the ice and gave everybody at the party something in common and interesting to play with. It was an on-site party so FUN was the name of the game and anything went. Quite a few couples went home successfully with others and even the ones who didn't still had a blast and spoke fondly of the party.

So, have fun! It's important for you and your partner, and everyone else involved. The more that you make having fun the point, the more that fun will follow.

Chapter 2: Maintaining a Healthy Relationship While Swinging

This chapter will cover the basic do's and don'ts for keeping your relationship healthy while you are dipping your toe into the shallow end of the swinging pool, so to speak. Jumping into the deep end with a new person or couple is not recommended, not until, as a couple, you have experienced enough to know what you do or don't want.

Take your time and get to know the lifestyle and the scene. Go only as far as you and your partner are comfortable with going each time. This process is different for every couple. The two of you will need to work together and communicate to know where you stand together. Swinging can bring a new level of satisfaction and honesty into your relationship if respect and boundaries are heeded and honored consistently.

Pay close attention to these do's and don'ts. They will have a heavy impact on how happily and successfully you swing.

#5. Do – Have a solid, healthy, honest, and communicative relationship before swinging.

Be sure that you, as a couple, have a solid and healthy relationship before you delve into swinging. There are many couples who swear that swinging has helped to save their relationships. More than likely this was because they were not being honest with each other about their sex lives, and the swinging lifestyle created for them a catalyst they have never had before for honesty and openness with their sexuality. Swinging can bring you closer together if your relationship is ready for it.

What will not bring you closer together is having a partner who already has jealousy or trust issues and expecting that going into swinging will fix this. A jealous and insecure partner will not be able to handle watching the other half of the team hitting on and partnering up with other possible "competition" without getting even more angry and jealous and may very well cause a situation or fight. That is because this person entered into swinging without covering the very basics – self-esteem and self-confidence.

Swinging couples without jealousy problems and trust issues will not have a problem when they see their partner hitting on or even having sex with another person. They know that they have no reason for being jealous or insecure. They are both sexual people and able to love their partners wholly and still have sexual freedom. They are honest and open with each other about their interactions, and often if not always include each other in their sexual adventures.

You need to know and trust your partner one-hundred percent, or be ready for a bunch of surprises. Know what types of people your partner likes, what their favorite type of sex is, and what their least favorite is. What sort of traits do they find attractive in others, both physically and mentally? Are they looking for emotional closeness to another couple or do they want unattached sexual trysts? Know what sort of toys they like and don't like and what sort of sexual games and fetishes they enjoy. Know what turns them off and on. Is your partner bisexual or straight? Have you just assumed they are straight when really they long for another woman or man?

Hopefully, as a couple, you know all of this about each other already. If not, then it is time to find this out. Set aside a series of date nights for just the two of you. Watch porn or cruise through various swingers' sites together. If there is an adult lingerie and toy store near you, take an evening to go shopping there and discover what sexual toys they sell. Explore every nook and cranny of each other and then some more. Sexual discovery of each other should never be relegated to just conversation, especially when there is so much fun to be had in the discovery.

Go to the adult book store or the regular book store and pick up some books on sex positions and games to play. Grab a bottle of wine or some beer and head home to delve into it together. Not only will you find out so much about each other, but you might also discover some new, interesting stuff together. Experiment with each other's fantasies, such as role-playing, using toys, BDSM, and other fetishes. Know what is on his/her curiosity list and yours; and what the absolute "no's" are for each other as well.

Playing and learning the ins and outs of each other's sexual desires will not only prepare you for swinging with other experienced couples, but also give you both an idea of what really makes each other tick. You will grow closer to each other and know exactly what you a looking for together when you begin to swing.

#6. Don't – Do this to "fix" a broken relationship.

While a swinger's lifestyle is fun and great for secure and confident couples, it is a recipe for disaster for those who are not already on the same page with each other.

Do not enter into swinging to fix a broken relationship. While swinging can certainly bring you closer together than you had ever imagined, it is not a replacement for therapy. It will not bring you closer together if you are already having major problems. Work through your major issues (whatever they may be) in private. Once are confident and trusting in each other as a couple again, then go ahead and discover swinging together.

If you are a couple who has issues and are looking for something new to draw attention away from the problems, please don't start swinging as a distraction. What will happen is that one of you, or both of you, will let an issue within the swinging setting start to drive the wedge further between the two of you, particularly if you two are having jealousy and hurt issues.

In relationships that have been heavily damaged and broken, it is easy for one of the partners to become jealous and angry when they start to feel that their relationship is threatened due to a newly established one with another couple. For a couple involves in swinging, it is imperative that they trust in their own relationship more than the new ones they are developing with other couples.

Some couples go into swinging thinking that perhaps if they go and play with other people together, it will spark their passion for each other once again. For some people it does, but for others it does not. I cannot emphasize enough how swinging is for couples who are confident in each other. If you have issues with your partner or yourself, then chances are watching them hitting on and having sex with others would only make these issues worse.

Some couples do go into swinging because they are not especially attracted to each other physically anymore. However, they still love each other and would prefer swinging over divorce or being unhappy. In this case, swinging in closed swaps may help.

There are many couples that swing because they spend lots of time away from each other due to travel or work. In these situations, they often grant each other permission to relieve their sexual and emotional needs with other people while they are apart from each other. As long as the couple is honest and happy within the terms of the agreements, there is no right or wrong way to go about swinging.

Do not to try to create a desire for each other out of being with other people or use the situation to create feelings which are lacking or not there at all. It will not heal anything but instead will further distance the two of you. Swinging holds no place for relationships in need of therapy and repair.

#7. Do – Talk about sex.

Many of us have heard the song "Let's Talk about Sex," by the group Salt N Peppa, and know the chorus by heart.

"Let's talk about sex baby,
Let's talk about you and me,
Let's talk about all the good things,
And the bad things that may be.
Let's talk about it.
Let's talk about sex."

Now is the time to talk about sex – lots of it and all aspects of it. After you have spent time getting to know yourself and your partner, it is time to discuss your sexual desires and expectations regarding the swinging lifestyle.

Know each other's limitations and have frank discussions as far as parameters between the two of you, both alone and with other couples. Be sure to cover all aspects of swapping, from full to soft swap to anal and group sex.

Discuss everything so that there are no surprises, and you have confidence and knowledge of how to act as a couple in any possible swinging scenario you might encounter. Also be sure to read through the terms in the beginning of this guide so that you know your terminology as an active swinging couple.

There is no set right or wrong way to approach swinging. It's all about doing what pleases you and your partner, as well as the people you choose to swing with. A happy convergence of sexual agreement and fun between consenting adults is to find common ground that both parties in the relationship are one-hundred percent comfortable with, and that the terms of playing are set clearly in the beginning. Failure to respect this could result in hurt feelings and mistrust later on down the road.

The smart thing to do is to discuss basic boundaries and sexual safety first. A good list of questions to discuss together would include:

- What form of protection will you use between yourselves and with other couples to prevent not only STDs but pregnancy as well?

- Will you allow bareback?

- Will you be having sex with other people together, in the same bed or separately, in different rooms?

- Are either of you into voyeurism or exhibitionism?

- Is the partner envisioning threesomes with you and other people or passing you around to others?

- Will you allow kissing on the lips, just oral sex and play, or full swaps with all four people involved in the swap sharing a bed and playing together?

- Who will be in charge of picking the couple that you swap with? Or will you both choose the couple together?

- Will you always swap with other couples together or will you be allowed to have random, spontaneous sexual encounters with other people separately of your partner?

- Will you grant permission slips and hall passes to one another?

- Will you consider bisexual swaps vs. straight swaps or bicomfortable swaps?

- How far are you comfortable with going with the other partner? How far are

you comfortable with your partner going with the other partner?

- What will your parameters be regarding anal sex? Oral sex? Group sex?

- Are you going to look for a closed
swingers group or are you willing to
swing more openly with any couple
you choose?

Cover all scenarios and know what to expect from each other and how to communicate
clearly to make sure you are both having the
best time possible.

#8. Don't – Assume anything about your partner or their expectations.

Don't assume that because your partner is
OK with you having sex with another person
during a swap that it is OK for you to have sex
with another person without them around.
This might seem like a bit of an extreme example, but I've seen it happened. A couple is
at a swingers' club, and then the wife is gone
to a play room with someone else's husband
and comes back freshly sexed while hubby

was looking for her. And surprise, surprise, hubby is now irate.

Do not assume that your partner wants to have sex with someone simply because they are talking to them and having a good time. Before you go into a club or party, you and your partner should know all aspects of properly interacting with each other in public and with other couples.

Establish a clear method for communicating approval or disapproval of another couple for a swap. If you allow open and closed swaps, then be sure to have a signal and communicate what type of swap you will be getting into with or without each other. Have a code for no and yes but one that is discreet and hard for others to figure out. (More on this in the next chapter.)

Make sure that you know what is going to happen and that both of you are comfortable with the other couple and the parameters that are in place. Cover all situations and possibilities before entering a club, party, or a date and that you have clear yet subtle signals to each other for yes, no, or a moment alone together. It is helpful to practice these signals to make sure they are not obvious. Having these tools, being aware and communicative, and never assuming anything will lead to informed and fun playdates for everyone.

#9. Do – Know each other's boundaries very well and discuss what would happen should these boundaries be crossed.

Discuss what boundaries will be in place for the both of you to keep the relationship happy, safe, and solid. Talk about what would happen should these boundaries be crossed by one of you, so you both know how to deal with the situation appropriately. Know what to do if the boundaries are not respected by another couple or partner of a swap, and how to deal with that properly.

It is important for you both to know how to handle situations gracefully while still maintaining your boundaries in a clear and strong way. What are you going to do if you have a "no kissing others on the lips" rule and one of the other couple in the swap began to kiss your partner on the lips? How will you stop this and still be able to maintain the flow of the situation? Or will you stop it?

Now this is where you must be careful. Some people who are involved in swinging, just as people everywhere, will not respect your boundaries. It is up to you and your partner as to whether or not to continue once the rules get broken. Perhaps it depends on the severity or the situation itself. Some couples have a no-tolerance policy, while others have a three-strike system in place. As long as it works for you and your partner, that is all that matters.

If and when you become involved in a scenario where boundaries are not being respected, approach it with calmness and class. Let's say the infraction that has occurred is the "no kissing" rule. The first thing that should happen is that your partner, who is being kissed, should respond by gently pulling their head away and say something polite like, "Ah, ah, remember the rules. No kissing on these lips, Sir.", and direct him towards other areas of the body that he can kiss.

If he attempts to keep kissing your partner on the mouth, it is going to result in ending of activities, or another, firmer request to stop. More often than not the first warning will be enough. Be careful of couples who do not respect the boundaries and rules, and be very wary should you continue to interact with them. Personally I would recommend avoiding these type of people.

#10. Don't – Push those boundaries. This will guarantee failure.

Everyone has boundaries and everyone has rules. It is also human nature to want to push boundaries and break the rules. Ever since we were little kids, we've had to fight this urge and overcome it. Here in the swinging lifestyle, there is no room for rule-breaking. This is how people get hurt and angry. Respecting the boundaries and following the rules help to establish fun and safe events for everyone. It is one of the most important principles in swinging.

Respecting yourself and your own boundaries, your partner's boundaries, the limitations you choose as a couple, and the parameters that other couples choose is paramount to a happy swinging experience. Disrespecting these boundaries is detrimental to the nature of swinging and will certainly cause negativity and bad situations.

No means no. This should be all that someone has to say if they are uncomfortable or do not wish to experience something. If you find yourself in a situation where you and your partner are uncomfortable, do not be afraid to say no or to put a new boundary in place. Be sure that you acknowledge and respect other people's boundaries in return.

Not everyone likes to do things the same way and that is ok. Find couples with similar boundaries or lack thereof to play with. Never try to convince someone to step out of their boundaries. It is awkward enough to have to discuss your most private sexual preferences with people who you don't know very well. It is even worse to have to defend your position or argue with someone about your sexual preferences and boundaries.

Pushing boundaries is rude, disrespectful, and unbecoming. There is no place for it in the swinging lifestyle. Always have respect for others' boundaries and follow those which are in place for you and your partners.

Chapter 3: Communication and Following the Rules

Communication is essential in the swinging lifestyle. It is critical not only between both members of the swinging couple but between all swinging couples and the leaders, managers, and hosts of any swingers' club or event. Not every place has the same rules so pay attention to the signs and the protocols that clubs, groups, or venues have posted. Know where to find them if they are not clearly posted. Follow and respect the etiquette as well as fellow swingers around you.

#11. Know the Rules

First and foremost, *know the rules!* Wherever you and your partner go swinging, be sure to do a bit of detective work so that you know the basic rules and expectations before you walk into the door of a party. Imagine showing up to the swingers' club and not knowing it was masquerade night, only for the doorman to not let you in for not having a mask.

Another example would be to arrive without your partner only to find out that the club won't let you in without a partner if you are a man. If you are a lady this is usually not a big deal. For men it is different. Doormen are going to assume that you already know this and will not always tell women who enter alone on the assumption that they already knew. Some elite clubs and parties will request to hold your cell phone while you enjoy the festivities and then your partner would have no way of knowing that you are standing outside calling her while she is waiting for you inside patiently or not so patiently. So be sure to enter with your partner always.

If the rules are not clearly posted, call or email the contact number or name provided. Introduce yourself as a new swinging couple, and let them know that you are interested in learning more about their club and the rules before you attend. Listen or read carefully to their response.

The rules that the club, event, or party has are just as important to follow as boundaries.

Rules can cover everything from dress code to code of conduct and designated areas of sexual play. To ensure the safety and fun of everyone, please make sure that you seek out these rules before you attend any event, even if it's a club that you have visited before. As mentioned above, many clubs won't let men in by themselves, so be sure to show up with your lady. Once inside you are free to roam around as you please separately, if that is what you and your partner agreed upon previously.

Know about the rules of play once you are inside the door. Just because a club is a swingers' club does not mean that there will be people fornicating in every corner. There are on-site clubs and off-site clubs. On-site clubs allow open sexual play and activity. Some have rooms for it while others have open play areas in the middle of everything.

Know what you are walking into so you don't do anything embarrassing for you or your partner. On-site clubs can offer faire that is as extreme as BDSM, with men and women being tied up and having sex in public, to more tame ones that have bedrooms, often on a separate floor, for the play to take place.

For the beginner swingers, it might be best to go to an off-site club the first time or two.

At these clubs, the couples meet to socialize and get to know one another before deciding on a separate location to meet and play at. Off-site clubs and parties offer a very inoffensive and safe environment for new swingers to get introduced to the lifestyle and setup a first playdate on comfortable terms, without feeling immediate pressure to swap or perform in front of groups of people.

Because off-site clubs do not allow open play and activity on their premises, the atmosphere is more relaxed and comfortable. It is easier for new swingers to be themselves. You get to really focus on having fun and getting to know other diverse couples in the club with you. Dance, laugh, and share a cocktail or two. Be careful, though, not to get too wasted, as this is rarely attractive to other people.

Online swingers' groups present a great way to communicate and have fun safely with other swingers from the comfort of your own home. It's also an excellent way to get acquainted with the scene and lifestyle without embarrassing or uncomfortable moments. It is important to know the rules and expectations for communication online as well.

Often online swingers' groups and clubs will have their rules clearly posted on a page on their group site. If it is not posted, message the group or the group leader and ask for the basic group rules. If there are not any group rules I would highly recommend that you consider looking for another site. At the minimum, there should be a "no means no" and an "18 and up" policy.

Rules can be complicated and explain everything such as the hierarchy and structure of the club, where you come in at the lowest rank and work up the ranks the longer you are a member, etc. On the other hand, groups can have rules as simple as have fun, clean up after yourself, and no means no. A good club will make sure that everyone knows these rules and follows them, and will utilize clear and concise communication to prevent any misunderstanding or bad situations.

#12. Communication between You and Your Partner

Communication is the foundation and groundwork for a successful and happy couple, and pertinent to the successful and happy swinging couple. You must communicate about everything and be willing to talk openly about subjects that society has taught us to keep as pillow talk. You must know about each other's sexual preferences and all the various aspects of their sexuality and fantasy fulfillment.

Once you have covered these bases, it is important to know how to successfully communicate with one another at whatever swinger function you are attending. Obviously you will both be mingling and entertaining yourselves with a variety of couples, men and women. As mentioned in the previous chapter, have very subtle signs for signaling yes or no, or attraction or non-attraction. A sign for "meet me alone" is never a bad idea either.

It is important for these signs to be discreet and subtle enough that they are not noticed or offensive to the couples around you. You can make it a certain touch on their arm or butt or a certain drink that you ask them to get for you. There are many ways to set up cute and unnoticeable methods to communicate with each other right in front of others without them having a clue that you are discussing anything at all. This will help to prevent awkward situations or having to explain in front of the people who you aren't attracted to that you don't wish to engage with them.

If you need to take time to discuss something that you forgot to clarify (or didn't think to clarify) between the two of you, take a moment to yourselves if it's unavoidable. Excuse yourselves for a smoke, a drink, or a bathroom break and take the time to make sure that you are in agreement with each other's desires and boundaries.

Go into each event with a game plan. Work together to look your best, and be one-hundred percent aware of the motive for the night. You can make the game plan anything you wish as a couple, from a mission to meet another couple to each of you going it alone to find the perfect someone to swap with. For beginners, the best game plan is to meet new people and have fun. Let the sex and more intense interactions happen naturally.

#13. Communication between Two Swinging Couples

When you do find a couple that you both want to play with, the next step is to clearly communicate about the boundaries and rules for both couples regarding play. I suggest that both couples talk about it together at the same time. However, many couples let the women or the men do the arranging and communicating.

So long as you and your partner have already discussed your boundaries and terms together regarding the swap, it is just fine to let only one party of each couple do the talking. This will be a fairly brief, though possibly brutally honest, conversation touching upon the parameters of the sexual exchange.

Things to discuss with the other couple may include open or closed, full or soft, bisexuality or bi-comfortableness, will you use condoms, who, if anyone, will take the voyeur and exhibitionist roles, and any others factors of importance. Covering these bases before play begins will help everyone involved to feel relaxed and ready to engage. Should anything arise out of the norm, "no means no" and there should never be any problem in relaying this message to anyone whom you are sexually interacting with and having it respected.

#14. Communication in Various Club Environments and Private Parties

Public clubs are clubs that are open to anyone in the general public over the age of twenty-one. Know if it is an off-site or an on-site club, and the rules pertaining to conduct and dress. We have already discussed this previously, but it is important to know the difference between an on-site and an off-site club.

When you are contacting an on-site club, be sure to find out if they confine sexual play to certain areas and VIP rooms, or if it they allow sexual interactions all over club. Be prepared to clean-up after yourself at any event or party as no one likes messy companions. Always pack and bring with you a little travel kit that include towels, wet wipes, condoms, lube, and any toys or lingerie you might need.

Private clubs are often invitation-only clubs. Usually they will have a night for new people to present themselves for consideration or allow guests from time to time, so always ask the person in charge. Private clubs may be held in either established buildings or venues, or operate out of the lead swinging couple's residence. They can include parties, events, or vacations taken by the club members together and with regularity.

Be sure to find out what type of event you are attending. The difference between a meet and greet and a costume party can be drastic, and you want to be prepared for the type of party you are walking into. Know who the host and hostess are, greet them, and bring a host gift when you arrive. Show up wearing your smiley face and have fun!

If it is an on-site costume party, then get your corset and condoms out and get ready to get down. If it is a meet and greet, then put on something slightly less risqué, get out there, smile, and get to know new people.

Above all if you have any questions or issues at all, it is best to talk to the management or host/hostess of the event to find out the best way to go about the issues or uncertainties. Do not just assume that because there is a bed in the corner that it is free for you, or that because you came across an empty room that you and whatever couple can claim it.

Just because you see someone "doing it" in the hot tub does not mean that it is okay. Different clubs and events have different policies about their rooms and play areas, so be sure to know them before you start to enjoy yourself too much and embarrass yourselves by breaking a rule.

Chapter 4: Meeting Other Swingers

Now that you know the basics, it's time for you to start meeting other swingers. Perhaps you've already had a few sexual encounters that involved multiple people. Perhaps you've even swapped partners with a friend. If so, that is great! You have a bit of experience under your belt and meeting other people who like to do the same thing shouldn't be too hard for you.

However, most people have never done something like this. How many people dream of being with two, three, or four lovers at once, but are hesitant to begin because sometimes pleasing just one partner is overwhelming enough? Having experience with multiple partners at the same time can be very helpful when you are starting to swing, but is not necessary. Everybody has to start somewhere, and the best place to start is by meeting other swingers.

Remember, swingers are out to have fun and get to know good people just like you are, so it's not as intimidating as you may think it would be. As a couple, and as an individual, you take bringing your sexual fantasies into reality into your own hands.

So, how do you meet other swingers? Where do they hang out? The answer is really everywhere, but there are some guaranteed places to start getting involved with other swingers. These range from social media groups and forums devoted to swinging online to clubs and groups to meet and join in person. Start to look and you will be surprised by what you find.

#15. Meeting Swingers Online

You have a bit of homework to do if you want to swing. The Internet is a great place to start meeting other swingers. Searching online is one of the best ways to get yourself started and to find swingers' clubs (all types) in your area. Suppose you and your partner live in a rural area far from any town or city that has an established swingers' club. The Internet can give you the ability to meet and play with other swingers via cam.

Below is a quick list that I've compiled for you. Use it as your starting point.

- Go to www.adultfriendfinder.com to search in your area.

- Look on www.craigslist.com to see if you can find any in your city. Sometimes, swingers will post about a gathering on Craig's list that is open to all. This is one of the easiest ways to find bars in the area that are swinger friendly.

- Visit www.swingersboard.com/clubs/ to find a club in your area.

- Find a club at www.swappernet.com/sn/groupsearch. aspx, you may need to create an account, but it's pretty fast and easy to do, plus, it's free!

- Go to www.swingersclublist.com and try to find one in your area.

- Check out www.kasidie.com and explore their clubs and events pages.

- Go to www.google.com and type in "Swingers' Club in YourArea" where YourArea is replaced with your actual location.

Take a bit of time to search for groups, forums, or clubs that peak your partner's and your own interest. Depending on the website or social media site, you can set up your profile and then search for other members in your area. Or you can set up a profile and search to join groups or established private swingers' clubs in your area or with similar sexual interests.

First, find yourselves a good Internet swingers' group. This will take a bit of dedication and involvement. There are many groups out there that were created for the sole purpose of promoting adult entertainment websites, or less tactfully, porn sites. If you have joined a lame group mostly used to promote porn sites, you will figure that out pretty quickly from the number of members who can't seem to spell or understand English. Remove yourself from the fake group immediately to save yourself from a barrage of promotions and spam messages sent through its boards.

Some of the more mainstream sites for swingers' profiles are AFF (Adult Friend Finder), Kasadie, and Lifestyle Tonight. Sites that tend to pan out some amazing private swingers' clubs, if you take the time to look, are Yahoo groups, MSN groups, or Google groups.

Look through the romance and lifestyle groups and you will start to find groups pertaining to a wide range of relationship and sexual interests and needs, including swinging. The more you take the time to look, the better chance you have of finding a group that will fit your needs, and ideally has fun, playful couples in your area.

As you read about various groups to join, find ones that are appealing to you. Take the time to get a feel for what the general nature of that group is and how it works. Put out a relaxed, open, and sexy attitude, and that is what you will get in return.

If you are on Facebook, Linked In, or any other social media site, you know how imperative it is to interact and be involved in order to get to know people and make connections. Likewise, in order to get good involvement and responses from other swingers on the social media site or within your group, be sure to interact with others on the site.

Introduce yourself right away but spend a few days treading water and getting to know the groups before you delve head-on into revealing everything about yourself. Be reserved on your interactions at first. Watch to see how others interact. Once you feel comfortable, jump in on the conversations and start some of your own.

As mentioned previously, pay close attention to the rules of the group. Take the time to read and know how the group works, as well as any rules they have and important information you should know before you can join the group. Some groups require you to come to one or two of their monthly meetings and get a feel for the group and your own chemistry before being willing to take you into the fold.

Meeting swingers online is a great way to get into swinging without having to worry about awkward situations or feeling uncomfortable in such new surroundings. It can also give you the chance to spend time with the other couple or couples in a group via webcam and chat to comfortably set up the parameters of your first swap. Once you are interacting with other swingers online for a while, you will quit being surprised by how many people actually do swing. It's not as rare as you think.

#16. Meeting Swingers at Off-site Clubs and Events

Meeting other swingers at off-site swingers clubs and events such as meet and greets is the perfect way for a couple to get into the feel of how to swing, especially without the added pressure of possibly having to perform in front of an entire club of strangers. After all, not everyone is an exhibitionist. Off-site clubs and events keep the pressure off of performing sexually, and put focus on having fun and getting to know the other couples. This makes them wonderful first experiences for new swingers.

Meet and greets are probably the best first experience for a swinging couple to have. The pressure is extremely light, and they often take place in a non-swinger establishment. Quite often, they are held by swingers' groups and organizations that are looking for new members, and there are usually quite a few other newbie couples to meet as well.

#17. Meeting Swingers at On-site Clubs and Parties

On-site clubs are a ton of fun and are recommended for the more experienced swingers. They come in all shapes and sizes, from kinky BDSM swingers' clubs where couples show up with one partner in a collar on a leash and the other holding the end of it, to more tame ones with play rooms for rent on the second floor. Know what kind of club you are going to and be ready to look the part and follow the rules.

Make sure that you come prepared for all the action. Have your game plan with your partner ready, as well as your confident attitude, big smiles, and knowledge of the rules for the night. See if you can find out extra information besides the rules from other swingers or reviews online before you go, so that you have more of an idea of what to expect.

Don't forget to pack up a decent play kit, including towels to clean yourselves up with, as well as condoms, toys, extra clothes, and anything else you might need for your play sessions. Pack it in as small and discreet a bag as possible. The less attention drawn to the play kit, the better, until playtime of course. Do not feel obligated to have sex with everybody or anybody if you and your partner do not find a couple that is right for you both.

If you are attending a private house party, prepare yourself for anything from very relaxed rules that include where you can have sex and what to clean up with, to more socially acceptable ones where clothing must stay on and no play is allowed. Be sure to arrive within thirty minutes or so of the start time of the party since once everyone has arrived, the host or hostess will often say hello and announce the rules of the party and what, if any, fun games or contests are going on that night. If you are late, be sure to find the host and get acquainted with what is going on as quickly as possible.

#18. Joining a Private Swingers' Club

Joining a private swingers' club is a wonderful and fulfilling experience for the couple who is looking to have a solid network of other swinging couples with which to make friends and have fun. They often meet a certain amount of times a month at very naked and sex driven parties, as well as hold meetings that pertain to the more business and platonic side of the club. There are clubs where all members are regularly tested for STDs and bare-backed sex between all members is openly allowed, as well as clubs where members set up and maintain their own boundaries as each couple prefers.

Be sure to know all about the club before you decide to join it, and find one that suits your needs. With the variety of clubs and groups out there, it is easy to find one to fit you perfectly. Clubs don't wish to bring in frictional couples, or couples who would not mesh well with their sexual style either, so don't feel bad in telling them no if it is not for you.

There are adult biker swingers' groups, BDSM swingers' groups, bisexual ones and more. Take the time to research thoroughly and know not only the rules but also the expectations and levels of commitment that they expect from their members. Some clubs have dues and mandatory monthly meetings. Some don't and maintain very casual rules and laid-back, open gatherings.

Also, pay attention to the structure of the group. Some are set up like a regular club with a voted-in president, treasurer, etc. Other private clubs run like a monarchy or with another hierarchical structure. Other groups function more like groups of friends that get together and play from time to time, and each member takes a turn hosting the sex party.

Regardless of what you are looking for, there is probably a group out there. Make sure that it is a good match for you and your partner before you commit. Find out if they ever host "meet and greets" to recruit new people for their group. If not, do they have any events or functions that would be appropriate for you and your partner to come and meet the group? Find out if they allow guest passes, or move on to another group.

Chapter 5: You Are at the Party, Now What?

#19. Take the Pressure Off of Your First Time Out

So, you, as a couple, have finally picked your first swingers' encounter to experience, and you are both just a tad bit nervous. Take the pressure off of your first time to a swingers' event by taking some of the heavy expectations out of the way. Be prepared to swing with another couple if you are ready for it, but focus on each other and having fun. It is much less stressful to leave the sexual mission at home and for the two of you to relax and get to know other swingers.

Use your first night out, and every subsequent night out, as a learning experience and a way to gain tools and knowledge for your next trip. Each time you go out, you will bring back new bits of etiquette of interacting with the swingers you have chosen to be around. Don't get nervous over the how to's or what if's of performing on your first encounter. The sexual encounters and playtime will happen comfortably and naturally so long as you stick to the guidelines.

As a couple, leave the expectations at home and arrive focused more on each other and meeting new people. That way the stress and social anxiety will become less of a factor, and the first time out becomes more fun.

#20. Breaking the Ice

How do you successfully enter an event or party and break the ice? This all goes back to having your game plan as a couple. Are you going to attack the scene together? Or will the two of you get to know people better on your own and then come back together to introduce each to whom you have met?

The first thing to do is to smile and introduce yourself. It is the most important part of breaking any ice. If you are new to a party or a club, find the hostess or host and introduce yourselves. Let them know that you are new and very happy to be there, and check to see if there is anything extra you should know that wasn't posted on their website or in the invitation.

If you are at a club, and not a private event, the person you will want to talk to and get to know first is the bartender. The bartender is a key figure at almost any event but most definitely at a club. Bartenders know everyone already and know how things work. Flash your smile, make sure to get their name, and tip well. Being friendly with the bartender often opens up the conversation for the people next to you at the bar, and allows for more ice to be easily broken as you wait for your drink to be poured.

#21. Smile

Smiling is amazing for you in so many ways. It increases your endorphins levels and actually makes you happier. It puts off a confident and happy energy, which in turn, gives other people a bit of a happy, confident energy.

Smiling also makes you look more approachable and easier to get acquainted with. People would rather get to know the person with a big smile on their face, who is laughing and having fun, as opposed to the person not smiling, looking shy, and quiet, or even worse, bored, aloof, and snobby. I've learned the hard way that not smiling can sometimes be interpreted in an almost offensive way.

So, be sure to smile and smile big. It will get you very far in the swinging lifestyle. It will make other people smile, help them to relax, and you will feel better yourself. I can promise you, if you smile at someone and catch their eyes at least three times, you are good to go to approach them at the bar or on the dance floor, with a compliment about their smile, dress, shoes, body, or whatever you feel most attracted to about them. Keep that beautiful smile on while you interact and mingle, and don't fake it.

#22. Dance

Most of the swingers' clubs have a dance floor and a play area, and there are some that have private rooms. I highly recommend the ones where you can dance, for many reasons.

- The event is more interesting that way. Even if you don't find someone to hook up with (which is always a possibility), you will still have something enjoyable to do!

- It loosens the mood and makes you more approachable.

- Dancing will lead you to meet more interesting and adventurous people.

Dance the night away and I promise that you will wind up knowing ten times more people ten times faster. Why? Do you ever notice that there is always a group of people watching the people who are dancing? No matter how many or few people are dancing, they are increasing their interaction with others as well as their likability and approachability. It's natural, it's social, and it's been a part of being human for thousands of years. There is something to feeling the rhythm and moving with the beat that helps us to feel connected to one another. The primal and natural motion creates comfortable situations that help to break the ice and get to know others.

Dance because it makes you feel good, happy, and more confident. Dance, move, and shake to the music. It will increase your energy level, your stamina, your hormones, and your happiness. Your smile will come naturally, and you will generate energy that draws people in.

Dancing gets you close to other people without words or awkwardness. Once you have spent some time on the dance floor with someone you don't know, you will find yourself introducing yourselves and getting to know each other better and with ease. Finding new people to meet and get to know is, after all, the point of this whole venture.

I've seen many hookups happen on the dance floor simply out of energy connections and sheer attractiveness. An added benefit to dancing is that it increases your stamina both in bed and in life. The more you dance, the more you have energy for other things as well.

Not only does dancing work for meeting others and hooking up in a swingers' club setting, but it is also a great setup for meeting new and open couples in some vanilla situations as well. Being sexy, confident, fun, and approachable are all traits that add excitement of your experience. Be sure to put on your boogie shoes, get down, and dance.

#23. Socialize

Get out there and be social, say hi, compliment someone's outfit or shoes, offer to buy them a drink, or ask if they want to dance. Have a few conversation starting tricks up your sleeve or even be willing to make small talks. I suggest sticking to easy, non-confrontational topics, and avoiding religion, politics, and other heavily charged, emotional, or highly debated issues such as abortion, family issues, or other uninteresting problems. Keep the conversation light, interesting, and playful.

Make a game with your partner to encourage the socializing and fun. Before you go into a party or club, make a bet with your partner to see who can get the most numbers or the most hugs, for whatever prize you agree on. Make it about meeting and getting to know the most people. The more people that you meet and get to know, the more likely that you are to find the perfect playmates and friends.

Don't just go to swingers' events for sex. Go to socialize in general. Practice will make you better. Get comfortable talking to the person in the elevator on your way up to the office in the morning or that quiet guy that works the counter at the gas station. See how many smiles you can exchange with strangers in a day and watch how your awkwardness fades away with more experience. Socializing is the precursor to more intimate swinging with other couples, so be sure to practice and enjoy spending time with others around you.

#24. Don't Be Shy

While not everyone is an exhibitionist (and that is ok!), it is important not to let your introverted side get the best of you at swinger's events. It is okay to be an introvert, just don't let it keep you from being open and social. It's going to be really hard to meet people and interact with them if you are pulling your best seventh grade wallflower impression. I've seen this happen at many events, and like most things in life, you get out of swinging what you put into it. If you are putting out quiet, reserved energy and behavior, then people will most often respond by giving you your space and following your social interactions and cues.

There are introverted people who enjoy swinging just as much as extroverted people do. It is important that you be willing to step out of your comfort zone in order to meet new people. If you are shy, be sure that you come out of your shell a little and talk to a person who is near you, or strike up a conversation with someone at the bar while you are ordering a drink. Make sure to smile a lot and don't cross your arms. Crossing your arms over your chest is a sure-fire signal that says "I'm uncomfortable, stay away." This is a very unwelcoming stance to take.

Grab a drink and a place to chill near or with other people. Do not pull out your cell phone and become immersed in that. Cell phones are a big "no" if you are out trying to meet new people face to face. They are almost offensive in some situations, suggesting that the people who are there are less interesting than the ones you are talking to on your phone. Sometimes, someone will suggest you put the phone down and start talking to you. If this happens, I suggest you put the phone away and strike up a conversation with them. However, most people will just leave you to your business on your cell phone.

If your partner is more outgoing, have a plan that involves the one of you making the introduction after the ice has been broken. The more outgoing partner can dance it up on the dance floor and meet some new people, while the more reserved partner stays back and gets to know a different set of people. If things go well, you might both meet new people! Maybe even the other half of the same couple. I've seen that happen before, too. With swinging, anything is possible. So don't be shy. Get out there and meet new people!

#25. Have Fun!

This has been covered already, but it cannot be stressed enough that it is important to have fun. Have fun with yourself, your partner, and others. Make having fun the goal of your night no matter what happens. Go out with an attack plan of smiling, dancing, and using your personality, charm, and beauty to have fun and meet new couples.

Be playful, crack jokes, and don't worry about all the little details. Worrying and stressing over the small stuff will ruin your night or playdate. The details and small stuff, when there is any to muddle through, won't last long. Usually a brief and respectful conversation about boundaries or a "no thank you, that's not for me" is enough to keep things moving in the right direction.

It is possible to not have fun at an event due to your own personal attitude, going into a situation with the wrong motives, or not being aware of the rules of engagement for where you are playing. Having a bad attitude or making a scene will not only make things worse, but it will also lead to creating a bad name for yourself. Your reputation, both as individuals and as a couple, will take you a long way. So be sure to leave a good taste in other peoples' mouths (in, umm, every way possible…) so that they want to have fun with you again and tell others how interesting you are.

Having a good reputation of being fun and easy to be around will go far in the swinging lifestyle. It doesn't take long for rumors and gossip to go around, but it takes even less time for the truth to spread. So be fun and respectful to all the couples you meet. Even if you don't wish to have sexual relations with another couple, it is important to have civil and happy communication. You can still have fun and be friends without sleeping with each other's partners. There is no reason for being rude to someone just because you don't want to sleep with them.

Obviously sometimes there are situations that are beyond your control and certain people just don't get along. This can cause a lot of friction and make things awkward, but only if you let it. If you are focused on having fun instead of any drama that might be occurring, people will be even more attracted to you and your ability to maintain positivity in negative situations and environments.

No drama makes for the best events and play dates, and knowing how to avoid this is a wonderful skill to possess. The best way to keep having fun is to just steer clear of people who create drama. Do not interact with others if you know it is going to cause tension or drama.

No matter what happens or where you are, go into swinging with an open-mind and a fun attitude. Keep the focus on having fun so that everyone else can have fun too. Fun is one of the sexiest things of all, and is a main part of the swinger lifestyle.

Conclusion

Now that you're prepared with the basic tools, get out there and start swinging! Spend some time with your partner and get to know more about the lifestyle. Begin putting together your game plan. Revel in your relationship, the new adventures, and things that you will learn about each other, yourselves, and those around you. Watch your self-confidence and your attraction to your partner grow as you explore together and learn more about the wonderful sexual adventures and fantasies that await you.

Converse honestly and openly with your partner and the other swingers that you meet to make sure that everyone is having as great of a time as possible. Keep an open-mind as the two of you meet new couples with a wide variety of styles and fetishes. Try new things together or separately, and discover the sexual limits to which you can take yourselves.

Maintain an awareness and be educated about the different situations you and your partner put yourselves into, along with the frame of mind to enjoy the event and have the best time possible. Know the ins and outs of and the rules of the different swinging situations. Always be respectful of the rules and follow them to ensure trust and confidence between all parties.

Together, as the two of you venture into this new journey of the swingers lifestyle, you will not only find that you grow personally and strengthen your own self-confidence and sexuality, but also that you can do the same for your partner and the other beautiful people you interact with. Always maintain honest and open communication among all parties to avoid awkward and unwanted situations.

Focus on letting loose, having fun, and getting to know new people and have new adventures. Above all, cherish yourself and your partner. Maintain a sexy attitude of fun and the rest will fall into place. The swinging lifestyle is for those who choose to respect one another and the people around them, and those who long for sexual adventures.

I hope this beginner's guide has helped you. Don't forget to check out the intermediate and advanced guides of this series. In the Intermediate guide, we will discuss:

- Importance of reputation within the swinging world.

- Practicing good ethics within the swinging world. (both public and private)

- Hosting the other couple and being gracious guests

- Swinging discreetly – how to swing without ruining your career and social reputation

- Play rough but play safe – how to take it to the edge without taking it too far.

- Exploring different fetishes within the world of swinging

- And more...

And in the Advanced guide, you will learn:

- Games for two swinging couples

- Games for more than four

- Fun positions for 2 couples (and 3...)

- Starting your own Swingers Club/Adult Lifestyle Group

- Throwing successful swingers parties and special events

- How to successfully bring in another party into a 2-person relationship

- Putting out ads for other couples

- Going on a swingers vacations

- Building a "sucsexful" playroom

- And more...

Happy swinging!